The Social Anxiety Cure For Women Workbook

Overcome Social Anxiety Disorder, Boost Your Social Skills & Enhance Self Confidence Without Struggling From Shyness, Depression Or Self Esteem Issues

PHILLIPA GOLDIE

Contents

Introduction

As a student, have you ever known the correct answer to a question that your professor asked, but didn't dare answer? In the workplace, did an inspirational idea flash across your mind that you thought your colleagues or manager would love, yet you didn't feel able to share it?

Have you ever spotted an acquaintance down the street and know that they'll stop to talk to you and ask you questions, so you deliberately crossed the road to avoid them so you don't have to make small talk? Not because you dislike them at all, but simply because you feel painfully embarrassed and awkward about trying to talk to them? Do you shy away from that social situation, with every ounce of your being, so that you don't have to face questions about how things in your life are going?

Do you feel awkward in social situations where you're introduced to someone new, unsure of how to keep polite conversation going and keen for any of your friends to come and rescue you, because your friends know and understand you and don't mind that you're quiet and shy?

Do you find small talk so difficult that you'd prefer people just not talk to you at all?

Do you feel misunderstood at times? Aware that people may perceive you as being a bit standoffish, rude, or abrupt, simply because it's all you can do to utter a few words? Because your face feels hot, your hands are sweating, your chest is beating uncomfortably in situations where you feel there's too many people about who you don't know, and you're not sure what to say?

If any of these scenarios resonate with you, you're in good company.

When I was younger, these types of things happened to me on a daily basis.

These events affected me physically as well as emotionally. I would have stomach pains, rapid breathing, and excessive sweating when I was put into a situation where I felt socially awkward. Afterward, I would make myself feel physically drained by overthinking everything that I had said or ways that I'd behaved. As I experienced these feelings every day, I just assumed that life would always be like this.

My shyness expanded into full-blown anxiety. I started to worry about the mortality of those I loved and I became very close to being suicidal. I'll discuss this more in later chapters.

This book, however, isn't my biography. It is written to help you overcome shyness and have a better life!

Through the easy steps in this book, you'll learn how to get rid of your shyness and be more social and able to express yourself freely.

Regardless of what type of personality you have, this book will make you happy to be exactly who you are! You'll feel confident that you can make friends - and brave enough to express your opinions when needed.

What is This Book About?

During the first section of this book, you'll learn more about yourself and work out what is stopping you from interacting with others and expressing yourself confidently. You'll learn how changes can occur, then start to contemplate how amazing life can actually be for you.

Throughout this part of the book, I will discuss my story and explain techniques that you can try out yourself in order to make meaningful changes to your own life. The purpose of this is to let you know that everything in this book has been tried out by me, my friends, and my family members. There is solid proof that it definitely works practically and not just in theory.

In the second part of the book, you'll learn various exercises that you can immediately put into practice to develop confidence and social skills. There is a great selection of hints and tips that you can use to create conversations and build friendships. When you use a tip, you may find that this gives you a boost in confidence, you feel like you're walking on air, and you're proud of yourself. Learn to love these moments - you deserve them! Other times, especially when you're first learning, you may feel a bit out of your depth and that it's a bit unnatural for you. That's OK, and is to be expected from time to time, but you're doing great and it will begin to flow better with time - I promise!

This book will use the phrase 'the true version of you.' What this means is that we can sometimes get taken up by fears and anxiety, or feeling judged, stressed, concerned, or as though we are unworthy or lack value. 'The true version of you' is when you naturally feel that you're accepted, content, grateful, appreciated, worthwhile, and calm. This is the person you would be if you didn't have any fears, any worries, or any beliefs about how others are viewing or judging you. This is you without a care in the world, able to just express every thought in your head clearly without any limits. This doesn't mean you'll turn into a brash, verbally-blundering oaf without tact or diplomacy - but simply that any time you want to speak socially, you are able to say what you want to express clearly and politely.

'The true version of you' holds no religious connotations. It simply means a state wherein you're happy and content with exactly who you are.

Chapter 1

The Prison of Fear

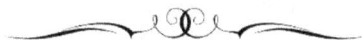

There's a quote by David Icke which says, "The greatest prison people live in is the fear of what other people think."

Lots of people have opinions about all sorts of things, but this doesn't make them an expert in the area. People are entitled to have certain viewpoints on matters, but it doesn't make them right. It is daft to worry about other people's opinions, and even more so to worry about speaking to others in case they don't approve of what we have to say.

Most people won't judge you or be as critical of you as you fear they will be. If people are, then it's quite possible they don't have a good understanding of you. Don't live in a prison of fear, worrying about other people's opinions.

When I was younger, I loved sports. Swimming was one of my favourites, because there's not much of a chance for conversation when people are mostly submerged in water. I did quite well with it. I also liked football, basketball, and baseball because they were all quite active. I became engrossed in the game, worrying about running and moving, rather than stressing about communicating with others. After high school, I chose to go to a very sports-oriented University.

I had, however, changed from simply feeling shy to experiencing a more extreme anxiety. I chose to avoid University dormitories. Instead, I decided to live with some of my high school friends. I had successfully managed to avoid mixing with large numbers of new people. I did participate in partying and I didn't study as much as I should have. I was drinking to avoid acknowledging the thoughts that were plaguing my mind. Drinking gave me false courage and allowed me to be more extroverted and chat with others. But I was living with fear - and drinking to excess. This wasn't good for my health, and I'll discuss this more in later chapters.

It is important to understand why we have the fears that we do. By understanding them, we can then more easily tackle them.

Fear and Shyness are Best Friends

Fear can be a sensible reaction. Fear is in our DNA from ancient ancestors, such as Neanderthals, who needed to know to run from woolly mammoths to stay alive. It was also important to remain part of a social group in order to have food, shelter, and to ward off predators.

In today's society, we still have fear. And some of this fear still relates to being part of certain groups - or feeling rejected from those groups. Rejection is a key aspect of fear. If we're rejected today, nothing will happen to us and we aren't in any danger. But we still associate rejection with loss and death. While rejection is unpleasant and upsetting, it isn't going to be a matter of life or death. It can just make us feel a bit rubbish.

In today's society, we feel rejection in many different ways. For example, we invite someone on a date, have to give a presentation, attend a job interview, or answer the phone. We fear that the person will say no to the date; we fear that the people we're presenting to won't like us or enjoy the presentation; we fear we won't get the job; we fear that people won't be able to understand us on the phone or will talk too quickly or quietly to be understood, etc.

This fear is inside us. If you're a shy person, you most likely have an overactive imagination. This can be a good thing and can make you very creative. But, it can also be detrimental to your well-being as you'll imagine the very worst-case scenarios and remember everything negative that has ever happened in the past.

But, you are in control of your imagination. You are in charge here. Instead of remembering everything bad that has happened previously, you can imagine yourself interacting well with people. If you have been worried about reacting in an interview, you can set the scene in your head of you walking in with confidence, shaking their hands, and creating a lasting impression of someone who is confident and in control.

When we're fearful, adrenaline kicks in and we're in fight or flight mode. We need to take the fight from the adrenaline and use it to destroy any fear.

Internal Critic vs. Living in the Present

When I was at College, I attended a drama class. I felt very daring attending a class that made me feel uncomfortable and took me out of my comfort zone. I did learn a really valuable lesson from the professor though that has helped me throughout life.

Each student was asked to give two 60-second presentations to the rest of the class about his/her background. On the first presentation, the person had a mirror that reflected their face for the entire minute. It was awkward for both the presenter and the audience.

When it was my turn, I was very aware of my appearance - my hair, my mouth as I spoke, etc.

When we each presented again, without the mirror, it was a far more pleasant experience for all involved - far more relaxed and fluid - even enjoyable!

When the mirror was there, we had a tendency to be focused on ourselves and worry about others' perceptions of us. We viewed ourselves harshly and worried about criticism. We were concerned with examining ourselves with internal, critical thoughts.

But, when we did not have the mirror, we were able to be ourselves, look at the audience and interact with them more freely.

If you spend too much time with your 'internal critic,' you're unable to live in the present moment.

If, when someone is having a conversation with you, you're constantly worrying about what your reply will be, then you're not truly listening to them. You're spending time with your 'internal critic,' rather than them.

Chapter 2

Opportunity

———— ✺ ————

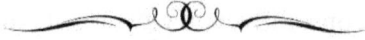

So, returning to the story of when I was at University and drinking way too much.

I woke up one morning, after a night of heavy drinking, and I felt really unhappy with myself. I played back everything I'd said the night before and was astounded at how stupid I'd been. (In reality, I probably hadn't said many silly things. I was just over-analysing and being hyper-critical of myself. Anyone else who had been there wouldn't have thought anything of the events at all). But, I spent the morning beating myself up about all the ridiculous things I thought I had said.

I felt like I needed a change of scenery, so I walked around the halls. But, all I felt was a sense of regret for everything I'd said the night before. I despised my actions and speech. I was also suffering with a hangover from too much alcohol. I took myself off for a walk.

I felt like I wasn't in control over how I was behaving.

I walked to a bridge and stood there for a long time,

watching the water below, and the thought truly crossed my mind: *What if I decided to just jump, and fall towards the water?*

I couldn't tell if I was still drunk from the night before. I'd never even thought about such a thing before. But, the worrying thing was that it was quite appealing to me; it would stop me thinking about all of the awful thoughts in my mind.

Thankfully, I broke out of this mood and realised that would be stupid. I took myself away from the danger of the bridge. I realised that there is ALWAYS something to live for, that life does indeed get better, and that my parents, family, and friends would be devastated if I killed myself. If you're ever feeling low and depressed or suicidal, consider family, friends, and people who rely on you (including pets who are dependent on your love and care). Think about seeing beautiful sunsets and sunrises, and of experiencing the sensation of the drizzle of rain on your skin. There are people who you have not yet met, but who will in the future impact your life and be so significant to you - and you to them - that you need to carry on living in order to meet them. There are things you can do throughout the course of your life that will make a true difference to others, whether that's volunteering, helping someone with words or writing, doing a gesture of kindness such as buying someone lunch or a coffee, or just listening. You are living your life for a purpose, even if you're not sure of that yet.

But, the very fact I'd even thought about committing suicide really scared me. I understood that I drastically needed to change things in my life to prevent myself from being in the same spot a few weeks down the line.

A few weeks later, I saw an advert for a self-help book by Vinny Guadagnino called *Control the Crazy*. I downloaded the book from Amazon and the stories in the book really resonated with me. I found that I just kept on reading and nodding in agreement with the situations that Vinny described. It made me very aware that there were other people who felt exactly like I did. I had felt alone, like no-one was experiencing what I did, and that I didn't really belong in the world. It was reassuring that other people had felt like me, and had gotten over that and were now living happy lives. If they could, so could I.

Changing my Mind

The book mentioned that every individual has 60,000 thoughts a day. I was astounded at this. I then jolted to Earth with a bump when I realised that three-quarters of my thoughts were quite negative and very anxious: worrying that I was shy; believing there to be something the matter with me; worrying about what I had said; wishing I was more confident; being envious of people who were, etc.

But then I thought, if Vinny, the author of the book, had felt just like me and managed to change, well then so could I! I simply needed to follow in his footsteps. There are many techniques I embarked upon:

- Yoga

- Meditation

- Compiling a 'thankful' journal

- Healthy eating

- Counselling

- Reading self-help books

I would also use visualisation techniques, imagining myself confident and no longer shy. It was great to be that free. The imagination is a truly wonderful thing. It's a bit like a call-out to the Universe about what you want. With time, the Universe has a great way of obliging and trying to get for you what you imagine. You clearly play a role in this too, but don't get too hung up about 'how' it'll happen, and trust that it will. If you imagine yourself being able to speak in social situations confidently and having a group of friends who are supportive, loyal, and fun to be around, chances are that in a short while, this will be the case.

I wanted to develop myself and have more power over my emotions and mind. I began to learn that this was definitely possible to do.

My life, from the outside, may have looked quite similar to how it previously had to other people. But I was beginning to feel different and better myself. A change was occurring.

Fulfilling My Abilities

Despite different socioeconomic backgrounds, opportunities, and education, each person can decide to shape themselves into whatever they want to become.

It may seem that some people struggle more than others. Some people may seem more confident, whilst others may seem more shy.

But, Tony Robbins gives good advice in his 'success cycle' of 'potential' – 'action' – 'belief' and 'result.'

It is possible for this cycle to perpetuate both positively and negatively.

For example, if you believe you only have the 'potential' to be shy, you may believe that you're shy, and this is how it will be all of your life. Your 'action,' because you believe you are shy, may be to avoid talking with new people or expressing yourself. The 'result' would be that you feel awkward and don't know how to behave socially around people. The 'belief' would be that you reinforce your own behaviour and say, "See, I told you so!"

Visualise the Changes you Want to See

You many get to a point which feels like your lowest ebb, and decide that you've had enough and need to make changes. You already have the answers to all your issues and problems. You need to identify them - then tackle them.

One key technique is for you to use visualisation to imagine how your future will be. Instead of having worrying, negative images, you'll create and imagine fantastic, positive ones. Believing that something is possible is more than half-way toward achieving it.

The runner, Roger Bannister, believed he could run a mile in less than four minutes. Prior to 1954 no one had managed to do this. But, he constantly visualised himself achieving this goal; and he did. People after that have done the same.

Allow yourself to be open to fulfilling your abilities. Allow yourself to imagine how it would feel being who you want to be.

This has been scientifically proven to work. If you spend 5-10 minutes each day visualising yourself as confident and chatting with people easily, it will become significantly easier for this to become a reality. It's like rehearsing for a theatre performance in your mind; you've already prepared yourself for how it will feel.

Chapter 3

Change

———— ⎯⎯⎯⎯ ⎯⎯⎯⎯ ————

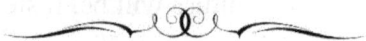

Approximately half a year after reading the book, *Control the Crazy*, my life still looked similar to how it had prior to reading it.

Because I'd started living in a healthier way, I was beginning to feel a little better. I wasn't drinking anywhere near as much, and I spent more time studying. These were small, positive changes that made a difference, but I was still uncomfortably shy.

At this point, I wasn't aware that there was going to be a change in my life.

As it neared the summer holiday, most of my friends returned to their families and jobs. Because I had failed a number of classes at University, I stayed in order to do resits, study, and continue working at a center on campus.

It dawned on me that unless I made the effort to make some friends, spend 12 weeks just watching reruns on the TV and playing computer games.

Then, the change occurred.

It seemed like a normal day. In my job, I was going

through my usual tasks; and then, almost like a rush of warmth through my body, I suddenly started talking to my colleagues and customers.

I was able to be cheerful and attentive, joke, listen well and respond accordingly; and I was beginning to develop friendships. It was the best feeling ever!

I didn't know what had happened.

Usually, after a conversation, I'd sit and analyse every aspect of who had said what. But instead, I just decided to go with it.

My shift at work went by at lightning speed, and it was soon nearing home-time. I didn't want to go home from work. This was the most fun I'd had in weeks.

When I did get home, it felt almost as though someone had cast a magic spell over me. I felt amazing. It was great having good conversations with people. I knew that this was a dramatic change and turning point in my life. It was going to be addictive.

The remainder of the summer was a great period of change for me. I viewed every single day as a chance to speak to someone new, learn something new, and overcome my shyness. I made so many friends in my resit classes and at work. These had been people who I'd seen plenty of times in the past but had previously been worried about chatting with.

I attended social functions, had a fun time, and managed to curb how much alcohol I drank. I explored the city where I worked; and that was fun. I approached summer by being accepting of suggestions and trying new things. I felt as though life was new and exciting; and I loved having good conversations with the people around me.

I enjoyed both work and my studies, and felt motivated and interested in both. There was a real transformative change in how I felt - from feeling shy, odd, not fitting in, and being perceived as the strange person in a group - to feeling that life is way too short to hide away or to worry excessively about other people's opinions. I felt that I wanted to make the most of every opportunity and to take every chance I could to talk to and learn from others.

I truly believed that I could get over being shy. And I felt that being shy had made me miss out on so many things in life up until this point. I was always a little envious of my father, who was a bubbly person who loved being around others and was the life and soul of every event. He had a good group of friends, who he often spent time with, and they really enjoyed his company. I had often wished I was like him, and it was only now that I started to think I could be.

Because I knew I was well on my way to overcoming the fear and shyness, I knew that I could tackle anything else in my life that was a fear. I figured that if I could overcome the anxiety that had dominated my life, then I could do pretty much anything that I set my mind to. Anything which in the past had been a barrier, I now brought to the surface and viewed as an opportunity to change in order to make myself stronger and better.

I had previously really wanted to study sports at College but did not have the faith in myself that I was good enough at it. I had also given up the one sport I was good at as a child for another, that I wasn't so good at. I went from being a strong swimmer to being a poor basketball player. I didn't look like a basketball player and I didn't play well. I spent most of my time senior year sitting on the bench.

But, I did know I had been good at swimming. Believing now that anything is possible, I couldn't help but ponder how good I'd need to get at it again in order to be accepted at College. It began to filter through my mind often and it was something I couldn't stop daydreaming about.

Your Change

So, you may be thinking that this is great news for me as author of this book. But, you bought this book because you wanted to stop being shy. And you may still be wondering how this will take place for you.

Well, whatever it is that you want to overcome, whether that is to become less shy, to improve how you communicate with others, or to feel freer to express exactly what you want to say without fear of other people's opinions, it is a 'change' that will enable this to occur.

Before we look further at how you can bring about this change, I want to emphasize - this book is about you being proactive and doing something to create change. If you don't do that, but simply keep reading self-help book after self-help book, attending seminars, and listening to webinars on self-improvement, you'll just spend your life searching for the answer. And you actually already know the answer and what needs to be done. Let's make this happen.

What is a 'Change'?

A change is that moment when you say to yourself, "Enough is enough. Something needs to change and be different from before." There is that old adage, "If you always do what you've always done, you will always get what you've always got." It works for many things in life, such as if you've always started a diet then a day into it, found yourself binge-eating packets of crisps and biscuits, you're always going to remain unhappy with the weight you are. If you're single, and fed up of being so, but never leave the house in order to meet someone new and never participate in any online dating sites, well then, you're probably going to remain unhappy and single. You need to make a change, whether it means that you eat more healthily and exercise if you want to lose weight, or that you go out more or join online dating sites if you want to meet a partner. If you want to make a change regarding your shyness, you need to take action, too, and speak more. There are lots of techniques in the second half of this book that will help you learn how to speak to others with ease; and I promise you that you will find it much easier than you expect.

It is highly likely that you have experienced change in your life. It could be that you've decided to give up smoking or stop eating chocolate. Or perhaps you've had a fall out with someone and later decided to let bygones be bygones and move on from that. Whatever that moment was, there was a change; and your life is different and hopefully better because of it.

The Strengths and Limits of Your Beliefs

In our own minds, we each hold beliefs about the type of person we are and what we think we're capable of achieving. To have this type of mental conversation with yourself doesn't make you insane - it's what everyone does. This type of belief system, though, shapes how you interact with the world.

This book will definitely give you hints, tips, techniques, and practical actions you can carry out which will enable you to become less shy and speak to people with confidence. But, if your belief system is constantly saying to you, "This is mumbo jumbo, and it doesn't really work," then you may remain a shy person - at least until you change how you think. Have faith that this book will work for you and I can 100% promise you that it will. It has worked for me; it has worked for my friends; and it's worked for other people who have read the book and followed the hints and tips and put them into practice.

The key difference between those who feel shy, awkward, and like they don't belong, compared to those who are confident, outgoing and fit in with people from all walks of life, is simply accounted for by the beliefs that each person has about themselves. My Dad, who is a very confident man, has a positive outlook on life. When he goes out, he expects that other people will like his company and find him interesting and funny; and they do. He never has any hesitance in this belief. He doesn't worry that people may think him silly or will be critical of what he has to say, whereas I previously had worried constantly about these type of things.

What are your beliefs? Do they boost your confidence and make you feel good about yourself? Or do they drag you down? Do your self-beliefs make you feel as though you are brimming with energy, or make you want to go to bed and just pull a big duvet around you? If your closest friend said the same things to you that you're telling yourself, would you still be friends with them? You need to learn to be as kind to yourself with your internal voice as you would be to one of your friends.

As mentioned earlier, the beliefs I had about myself were: I lack confidence; I'm odd; I find it hard to make small talk; I feel self-conscious and in the way or out-of-place; I don't fit in. I'd worry about talking in case everyone thought my ideas were ridiculous. Whether these were true was entirely my choice. My beliefs became true by me acting them.

To change the beliefs I held about myself, I used a technique learned from meditation. I would internally examine all the beliefs and thoughts I had, in little cloud-shaped bubbles. If the thought was a good thought and boosted my self-esteem, the cloud bubble was allowed to stay. If it wasn't a good thought, then I was let the cloud bubble float away out of my ear.

We become what we think of ourselves.

Instead of focusing on the negative: "I don't want to be shy," you need instead to focus on what you do want. Saying "I don't want to be shy," almost works as an affirmation that you're a shy person and you believe it. Instead, try changing the way you think to, "I want to be bubbly and confident with lots of friends." This is a much more positive cloud to have in your head, and to keep there, without it needing to float out of your ear.

This isn't just wishy-washy, self-help, positive-thinking rubbish. It works in an ingrained psychological way.

In a similar way to how our beliefs shape how we view ourselves and others, how we feel energy-wise has an impact on our real-life experiences.

If you feel shy and timid, you'll talk yourself out of acting confidently in conversations.

We will use the analogy of a thermostat for the way you think. Now, let's assume that over time, you have become comfortable with the thermostat set to 72 degrees. Each day, your temperature will be affected by good things that make the temperature increase, and bad things that make the temperature reduce. But, with time, you find your way back to the 72 degrees where you're most comfortable.

When you're trying to be less shy and need greater energy to do this, you'll need to adjust your thermostat to around 75 degrees, initially. This will require effort on your part because you'll be unused to it being so warm, and you will feel a little uncomfortable until you are accustomed to it.

But what you need to note is that it's you who is in full control of the thermostat.

You can control your energy using your body. You can change how you feel by how much you move and how active you are. We all know that we can tone our bodies, develop muscles, and create endorphins when we exercise.

It's not necessary to exercise directly before engaging in conversation. But, doing some exercise each day will make your mind much more active and open, too. If we mentally try to persuade ourselves to do something, it can be really hard to get motivated. But, if we physically move ourselves, it will give more energy and positivity to our minds too, and give us much more willpower and determination.

You need to start monitoring your energy levels. When they reduce, you need to find a way to increase them, as it happens.

The Optimum Moment

Your 'change' will occur when your mind is energized, active, and open, and when your beliefs are positive and you're mentally excited about what the future holds. This will be your optimum moment, when all the pieces fit together. Something will trigger this, and it can work in odd ways. Sometimes it can be when things have gone well and you're encouraged to push yourself to move onto something new. At other times, when things seem bad, it can be the catalyst for change. It can be a point of, 'Something needs to change now,' or, 'Things are at rock bottom. There's only one way to go from here, and that's up.'

This optimum moment of transitional change will occur one day. You dictate when this change happens. You can decide to make that change right now. Or, wait until a year down the line when you decide to change then. The decision is entirely yours. But I would encourage you to make the change as soon as you feel you possibly can, because your life will be so much better. The very first time you apply one of these techniques from the back of the book, you will be glowing with pride in yourself for days. And this glow will portray you as being happier, more confident and content, and will attract more people to you.

The very first time I tried the technique was when I went to a music gig with my partner. The musicians from the gig, after performing, mingled with the audience. I'd seen a musician and wanted to talk to him - and I plucked up the courage to do so. I wasn't awe-struck. I spoke sensibly to him about his previous occupation and managed to end the brief conversation with a polite, "It's been nice to meet you." But the fact that I'd plucked up the courage to do this made me smile for days afterwards, every time I thought of it. I could see the look of surprise on my partner's face when they saw I was talking to someone, because I was usually so shy. My partner even took a photo of me chatting. I was pleased when I saw in the photo that I was holding my hands in an appropriate place as I chatted, and I was smiling and looking interested. All of these aspects of poise will be discussed later in the second half of the book. I did it - and so can you.

Chapter 4

Growing Yourself

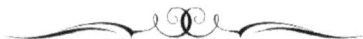

So far, the book has discussed changes that you'll make and actions you'll take to become less shy. Change happens, regardless of whether we want it to sometimes. But, the key thing here is growing yourself so that you're more who you should be, who you were meant to be, and who you would be if you were free from the many constraints that society places on us and the barriers we have built up around ourselves.

There is nothing wrong with you at all. And don't for one moment think that there is. This book isn't about you 'changing' who you are as a person because there is nothing wrong with with you as you are. It's about you growing and developing as a person to become the best version of you that you can be.

When you grow into the person you are, you'll become friendlier and enjoy conversing with others. And you'll be prepared to be sillier and less concerned about letting your reserved barriers down. You'll feel free to express what you're passionate about - your interests and hobbies. You won't be shy and quiet about these or worried that others won't find these interesting. When you talk about things you're interested and enthusiastic about, this excitement will rub off on others. If you speak quickly, timidly, or with reservation, about a topic, people won't find this as stimulating as someone who can barely control their excitement. You need to understand your fears first of all, and you need to experience that instant when you'll change.

When that summer was approaching its close, I decided to make some plans for the future. I dared to imagine what it was in life that I desired, and this was a new thing for me.

I wasn't sure of exactly how all this would occur yet. But, what I did know was:

1. I wanted some sort of new experience

2. I wanted to do swimming at College

3. I wanted to live in a warm environment

I was very excited and hopeful - and my answer came to me. I decided to move away from home and go to a school in Southern California. It was like a clean slate for me; a brand-new start. I was free to create a life for myself, exactly of my own choosing. This was what I wanted, and this is what I did. I was determined that this should be my course of action and I did everything I could to make it happen. Just four weeks later, I'd packed all my belongings in my case and was ready to set off in my car on my next life adventure.

Liberating Being Me

Happiness.

Happiness and contentment ran through my veins as I drove for two days to my new life in Southern California. It was a wonderful road trip. I enjoyed driving; I had the car windows open, a breeze blew in, providing some relief from the heat, and I had my favourite music on. It made me feel as happy and carefree as I'd been as a child.

As I drove, the concept of a 'clean slate' really appealed to me. No one knew me in Southern California. I didn't have any excess baggage, with people perceiving me as the 'shy one,' or the 'nerdy one,' or the 'odd one who never really fit in.' If you're in a place where everyone knows you, it can feel harder to suddenly decide to dress or act differently, because you'll have people seeing how different it is. However, they would soon get over it and adapt to the new version of you. Moving isn't always the answer, or the only option. In Southern California, I was free to create my own identity exactly as I chose. I could decide to act and behave exactly how I wanted to there, and people would just assume that's how I'd always been. I was thrilled, and it just felt amazing!

Have you ever felt like that?

It is a wonderful thing to realize that you can create this clean slate, this new start for yourself at any point you want to. You don't have to move schools or locations to make it happen. The only thing you do need is to make the decision to change and have the determination to stick to it. People around you who know you may be a little shocked or surprised upon the first instance of you suddenly becoming chatty, confident, and outgoing. But if you keep on doing that, this will become the new perceived impression of you. When someone is confident, it can be a little disarming because it gives a person poise and shows contentment and total happiness, but it's also very appealing and nice to be around. It can put others at ease, too.

At University, I settled into my accommodation, then I immediately became involved in mixing with the people around me. Some of this was driven by anxiety. I was more concerned with not having a group of friends than people disliking me. So, I tried really hard to make friends wherever I went.

Within just 2 weeks of being there, I gained a position on the swim team, joined the student government, and gained employment working on the reception desk of the student accommodation. My key motivation with all three of these was to make friends and enjoy myself as much as I could. That's a really nice approach when you start anything new, whether that's a sport, a group, or a job. Wanting to meet new people and find out about what they have to say and the things you can learn from them, and wanting to having fun and enjoy yourself is a very positive way of life. You'll see the best in people, be friendly, smile, and joke; and you will attract all this back to you.

You'll be a fun person to be around and you'll find yourself invited to more social functions. It's a circle whereby you'll constantly expand your group of friends.

I pretended that I was a social, outgoing person, and had always been; and it became reality. It was very natural and didn't take any effort.

As it happened, I was only able to stay at that school for a semester, so I had just three months there. This was because I couldn't get the money to cover the fees going forward. But, I shall always look back very fondly on that time as being significant in my development.

During that time, I made friends who I'm still in contact with today. I achieved my dream of being a college athlete. I was no longer stilted by my fears or anxieties, but faced these head on. I was very happy and at ease with life.

One of the key things that I took from this was that I discovered I could be enthusiastic and passionate about things in a way that I never realised I could be. I would never have realised that I had this kind of drive in me if I hadn't pushed myself into a place beyond my comfort zone.

If you want to be a confident person and achieve certain aims in life, at times you will need to step outside of your comfort zone and move into places where you stand the chance of rejection. But you will certainly develop and grow from your experience.

There's a book called *One Minute Millionaire* wherein the author, Robert Allen says, "Everything you want in your life is just outside your comfort zone."

When you push yourself to a place beyond where you're comfortable, you may feel a bit odd and awkward at first, but this is the place where magical things happen. It's similar to when you're brave enough to enter the sea. The water may feel cold at first, but you soon acclimate to it and enjoy splashing around, it feels vibrant and exciting.

This is similar to stepping into a new area out of your comfort zone and becoming closer to your true self.

One evening a week, I was asked to give a small talk about my experiences by the Student Body President. The idea initially terrified me - which is why I decided to go ahead and do it. I was out of my comfort zone and I realised this was good for me.

As I gave my little talks each week, I shared information about deciding to move to California. I had never felt more alive than I did when giving these talks, and I realised that I was motivated by my ability to inspire other people through my stories.

Previously, if anyone had suggested that each week, I'd standing in front of a group, confidently talking about myself, I would have thought they were completely deluded. This would have terrified me in the past. But, I knew the group was friendly and genuinely had an interest in hearing from me, so I thought I'd give it a go. With time, upon giving the talks, I felt more and more confident. People listened; they were interested and would ask questions afterwards. People thanked me for the talks and told me how much they'd enjoyed them or how they'd helped them.

It could be that you already have a very clear idea about what you want to do with your life. Or, you may feel that you're just going through the motions of life, with no clear idea of direction. You may feel stuck in a rut, like everyone seems to be making progress in life - bar you, that time is just standing still for you. Being stuck is a horrible feeling, because you find it hard to see how you're going to get past this brief phase, and how life will be any different from this in the future. But, you will. Life will get better; this is just a blip.

If it is simply your shyness that you feel is preventing you from being your true self, then this needs to be worked on right now. You need to let the person trapped inside your shy exterior escape and be free. You have the power and ability to do this. I know; I have been exactly where you are right now, and I've escaped. And it's the best thing that has ever happened to me, which is why I'm encouraging you to do the same.

Think briefly of your very worst-case scenario...

Imagine you're in a bar and don't know anyone at all. Imagine you pluck up the courage to go up and chat with a group of girls and say, "I wondered if you'd mind if I joined you for a short while. I don't know anyone here. Would that be OK?" In the worst-case scenario that the girls sniggered and said something like, "Actually, no. We want to be on our own," what's the worse that happens? You may feel that they were a bit rude. You may feel a little hurt and a bit rebuffed. But, IF that happened - and that's a big 'If' - that says more about the group of girls than it does you. It shows they're not very welcoming and not very friendly; but, it says nothing bad about you. You've been polite, open, honest, and friendly – and those are all really good qualities. If they giggle, they may be doing so out of awkwardness or immaturity, or they could be just being mean. It still doesn't say anything bad about you. Whilst you may feel slightly rejected… That's the worst that happens. You don't die! You live another day. You dust yourself off and realise this is actually a good thing. You've learned quickly that they're not your type of people. You move on from them, ideally that very same night, until you meet people who are better aligned with you. I actually think the chances of being rebuffed by a group are very slim. Most people, if approached in the right way, will welcome you into the group, make introductions, and do their best to include you in conversations and make you feel at ease.

Making the Most of Your Abilities

Your aim is to be more confident with a bubbly personality. To start this, you need to believe that you will be more confident and visualise yourself being more confident and less shy. I'm one hundred percent positive that you have hidden abilities and expertise that you may not have even realized. I believe that every single person has a special skill or ability, something that they're talented at, that makes them stand out from the crowd. Everyone has strengths - things they're good at. If you're unsure what it is, start by thinking about what you most enjoy doing. Generally, people enjoy the things that they're good at because it comes naturally to them.

One of the key ways that your life can be more exciting and special to you is to set yourself aims and decide to make a change.

If you spend too much time dwelling on how shy you are, you'll trap yourself with negative self-belief and won't be able to move from that position. You'll think that you're shy, and therefore will act in a shy way, avoiding conversation, not chipping in with opinions but rather keeping them to yourself. You'll avoid social functions and will miss out on a lot. When you believe something about yourself, you then tend to act in this way. It's a self-fulfilling prophecy. You'll become stuck and stagnant in life.

What you need to do instead is focus on how you'd like your life to be; the universe and our own minds will find a way to make this happen. When you're thinking about an ideal world, if you could be anything, do anything, and have life exactly how you consider to be perfect, what do you see? Now think about it again, but ensure that you pack the image with as many details, colours, and textures as possible. You need to really bring this daydream to life in your mind. Make it as vibrant as and as realistic as you can. Think often about this.

My life changed dramatically once I started to talk more confidently to others. I followed a route of acting how I wanted to behave and trusting that this would work; it did. I know that this can work for you, too.

Setting Great Goals

Toward the end of this chapter, I'm going to encourage you to really talk to your inner child and allow yourself to dream with no barriers at all. Absolutely anything is possible in this exercise. You don't have to be bound by what is 'realistic'; just simply dream. To truly get inspiration and be inventive and creative, you have to dream big without any limitations. Many people who have created new inventions did so by allowing themselves to dream big with no limits, then worked out later how the dream could be achieved. Many people who have started new businesses again allowed themselves to dream big initially, then worked out a little later what was immediately feasible and what would have to wait until a little later.

This is a wonderful, enjoyable thing to do. But

firstly, you need to ensure that you're in the best possible mood for this to work as well as it can. You need to be feeling energetic and filled with enthusiasm before starting this task. If you need to do some physical exercise in order to get yourself pumped up, and the adrenaline running, then do so.

The next thing to do is to take a notepad and a pen and write out 50 goals! These can be any type of short-term or long-term goals to do with health, fitness, hobbies, your career, spirituality, finances, or any other goals you may have.

Because the key aim of this book is for you to be more social and confident, that should certainly be one of the goals you include on your list. So, your aims could include being more confident, less shy, able to speak in front of groups, able to express your views, and to be a person who is content with their life and does not feel like they're being held back in any way.

Try not to stop writing goals until the 30 minutes is up. If you have more than 50 in that time, that's great! If you don't yet have 50, then take a bit more time until you have reached the 50 mark. I swiftly managed to write around 40. The last 10 were a little harder for me to think of - but, I soon got there. This is a great exercise for focusing your mind on what is important to you. You may find on your list some goals that you 'think' you should have, either because this is what your family expects of you or what society thinks should be goals for people. But later, when you come to prioritise those goals in the next step, do ensure it is YOUR goals that you're prioritising - what YOU really want, not what is expected of you by others.

Next, from your list of 50, ensure you have the top 5 goals that you're most passionate about. When you're enthusiastic and excited about your goals, that lets you know that these are the correct things that you should be focussing on in life. At least one of these goals should be a goal that relates to being less shy, more confident, and more social.

The next step is that you need to search the Internet or magazines to find pictures that represent what success in these goals looks like to you. So if, for example, one of your goals/aims was to dress better, you could find images of the type of clothes, shoes, and accessories that you'd like to wear. Over time, finances permitting, you can gradually add items to your wardrobe so that you can make this a reality.

If your goal was to have a nice circle of friends, you could find images of groups of friends enjoying various activities together, such as: meals out; meals cooked at one another's homes; trips to the theatre or cinema; game nights; day trips to new places; BBQs in the summer; evenings by the bonfire; Halloween or Christmas together; baby-showers; cafes for tea and cakes; playing golf; attending gigs; weddings; walks etc. - whatever it is that you like to do, and would like to spend time with friends doing.

If you're determined to make friends and have a nice social circle, you will. Remember though that friendship takes work. You can't always wait for people to contact you to ask if you'd like to do something. If they have contacted you though, try to make time to spend time with them. Everyone has busy lives, juggling work and family commitments and various other activities, but try to spend time chatting, have cups of tea/cake, have a pint at a local pub, or a game of golf, etc. Check in on your friends from time to time, to ask how they are and invite them places.

Don't be hurt or take it to heart if they don't want to go where you invite them, or aren't able to. They will also lead busy lives and be juggling many things. What you can do is try to have a fairly open invitation rather than to a specific set event, where you say, "Would you be free to meet up any time from X date onwards? I can't do X, Y or Z, but I'm free at other times." This gives your friends a clear chance, which is as open as possible, to check their diaries and schedules and find a convenient time. If they're not free, then ask them to suggest an alternative date/s to see how that works for you. It's nice to have dates to meet up with friends scheduled for the future as it will give you something to look forward to. And it's always nice to chat with others and find out about their lives and learn something new.

So, these 'ideal' and 'perfect' images you've found of how you'd like your life to be, taken from either magazines or the Internet - you need to bring these images to life and have daily reminders of them. You can either print these images out or create cards with them to make a vision board that you can look at to what you want in the future. The brighter and more colourful the better, as it's easier to visualise. I like the idea of a vision board, and it works well for me personally, because often some of your goals are linked and it's nice to be able to cast your eyes over all your goals at once and to have these easy to see.

The next step is to attach an affirmation to each of these images, as though you have achieved the goal and you're living with that achievement every day. The more detailed you can be about exactly what it is that you desire, the easier your mind will find the answers and make it happen. Use confident language in your affirmations and say things such as, 'I am outgoing, sociable, and bubbly with lots of friends.'

You need to look at these goals every day. You need to believe that they are already true each time. You need to use your imagination to put yourself into situations where you act out what would be your desired result and prepare yourself like a dress-rehearsal for when this is true in your day-to-day life. When you set a goal, it can often be more about the journey to the goal than the goal itself. In the process of reaching your goal, you become a different person. Every single time that you look at the images, and read the affirmations connected to them, you'll feel enthusiastic about imagining that situation as though it was a reality. When you read your affirmations, ideally aloud, be as energetic, passionate, and brimming with enthusiasm as you can. Every day, have your vision board or notecards in sight so that you see them, especially first thing in the morning and before you go to bed, and have these images firmly in your mind.

You may not understand currently why you're working on goal setting when this book is about you becoming less shy and more sociable. It's sensible to ask. But, like a smoker who finds it difficult to cease smoking until they partake in a new habit that distracts them from smoking, you will not overcome shyness until you become so focussed on working towards your aims and goals that you'll be too busy - and too involved in and passionate about your goals - to care about being shy.

This may sound odd, but I have lived through this experience and know it to be true. I know that if it was the case for me, it'll be the same for you, also.

You need to have goals and look at them daily.

Chapter 5

Be Realistic and Honest with Yourself

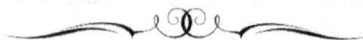

———⟨❀⟩———

This is the point of your life where you need to be realistic about yourself as a person. In order for me to get to the point where I decided to overcome my shyness, I spent a long time writing in a journal, read self-help books, and had regular meetings with a counsellor.

Each time I met with a counsellor, it gave me a feeling of relief and freedom. It was only with the counsellor that I felt comfortable sharing information about myself that I hadn't shared previously with my closest friends and family. It was important for me to speak with a complete stranger, because otherwise I may have been worried about being so open and honest and may have not wanted to hurt my friends or family's feelings. Therefore, I wouldn't have said everything that was on my mind. It's great to have the ability to speak freely, and be listened to, in a completely non-judgemental way, with no fear of upsetting someone.

Right here and now, let everything out!

How to Express Yourself Freely

2 key ways that stand out are:

1.   Having professional counselling

2.   Writing your feelings in a notebook

If you don't feel that you want to talk to a person about how you feel, then writing your thoughts will work just as well, only it's cheaper and you can do it from the comfort of your own home, at any time that is convenient to you!

Set a stopwatch for half an hour and write anything that is on your mind. Absolutely anything. Do not stop writing until the 30 minutes are up. I would advise you to do this on notebook paper using a pen or pencil, rather than typing these electronically. Try to do this every single day - but at a minimum you should be aiming for three times a week.

When you maintain a notebook or journal of your thoughts, feelings, dreams, impressions, and experiences, it's a great way to keep track of them. It allows you to organize them and become clearer about them. This can lead to dramatic insights, which can have an impact upon future thoughts and behaviour. A journal should contain a description of what has happened as well as your thoughts and musings about it.

What is great about keeping a journal is that it's only you who will read this. You're not writing for an audience, so it doesn't have to make sense to anyone but you. You can ignore any spelling mistakes, grammatical errors, any issues with your order, or whether it is easily understood. You can be one-hundred percent open and honest and not worry about hurting anyone's feelings or making a fool of yourself. You can be as creative as you want with it. If you are writing content that could potentially be misunderstood by family members, then try to ensure you keep your journal hidden away somewhere safe when it's not in use, so that it isn't easily accessible.

Your journal can be used as a key way of understanding yourself. Life today is busy and fraught with pressures. A journal gives you an opportunity to slow life down, think about it, and work out how you feel about things. Itl acts as a way for you to talk to yourself about what is important to you. Doing this lends strength to who you are as a person, and it allows you to deal with whatever life throws at you in a more positive way.

There are some general guidelines about keeping a journal that you may find useful to apply in order to lend it some structure:

1. Make a note of the date each time your write; it will allow you then to have a perspective of time as to when things happened and how you were feeling.

2. Write in the journal exactly when you feel like it. Do try to think about how you're feeling and write this down. Don't make yourself write if you're not in the mood; instead have a break from it until you

are. With this in mind, it can be beneficial to have a blank notebook rather than a diary. With a diary, you can feel pressured if there are lots of blank days, whereas if you're dating a notebook as and when you want to write in it, there are never any 'missing' days.

3. Be truthful at all times. There is no point in keeping a journal if you're not going to be honest. You're not writing for an audience; you're writing for you!

You may find it useful to have a set time of day or night that you write, when you won't have any interruptions. You may decide to write a certain number of pages or for a certain amount of time. But the key thing is to express everything you're feeling. I personally find that a set amount of time, with a timer set, is useful to me. Again, I'm not tied to writing for any longer than I want. If I chose 3 pages, some days I'd fill that quickly; other days I may agonize over writing them and it'd take forever. But, if I set aside a timed amount of 20 or 30 minutes a day and write as much as I can in that time, whatever I can get done is always acceptable to me. There's no target that I've missed by not having completed the 3 set pages. If I write 2 pages in that time, great. If I write 2 paragraphs, that's also fine. This is meant to be therapeutic and helpful to you, not something that you feel bad about, or beat yourself up about for not meeting a target.

If you are ready to talk to a counsellor, then try to find someone local. If you're in an educational establishment, there is often have a counselling department connected to them. They are trained to listen and gently guide you to make decisions. A counsellor will never tell you what to do or give you advice; that's not their role. But they will listen and help you to reach decisions that are right for you based on what you decide. You are in control.

This first half of the book has focused on creating the right mental state. In the second half of the book, you will learn tips and techniques that will allow you to have more control over your life.

Chapter 6

Choose Your Friends Wisely

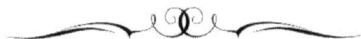

Often when we're growing up, people may try to guide you to stay away from certain people by saying that they were a bad influence, whether that's your parents or guardians, siblings, or other friends. They may have tried to encourage you to hang around with others because they seemed like nice people. You may have ignored their advice and done your own thing.

But, their advice was probably sound. There's a personal development expert, Jim Rohn, who states, "You become like the five people you spend the most time with. Choose carefully."

Have you thought about your close friend group?

These 5 people who are closest to you will either make you become a more social person who handles themselves with confidence, or else reinforce your shy, reserved behavior. It's inevitable that you will behave like the people you are closest to.

It's not their role or duty to behave in a certain way; you chose to be their friend. They will behave in the best way that they are able to.

People do, however, change over time; and so do friendships. If you have 'friends' who end up making you feel down, depressed, or fed up, then look closely at your relationships with them. If you have friends who frequently drag your mood down, consider carefully if these are people you want to spend a lot of time with. If they're not, then start to reduce the amount of time you spend together. You don't have to dramatically break off friendships - it doesn't have to be all or nothing - but you can spend more of your time with people who make you feel better. Life is short; you want to spend as much of your life as possible having fun, laughing a lot - real belly-laughs with tears streaming down your eyes - and looking back on fantastic memories of time spent in good company.

You can be very fond of someone, but still aware that if you spend too much time with them, it will drag your behaviour and activity into a bad place where you don't want to be. For example, if you have friends who drink heavily and party hard, then you may want to still be friends, but not spend every night of the week with them. Or else, if you're studying, you won't get good grades, and you'll probably damage your liver! Distancing yourself from people can be tough, but effective.

I'm not suggesting either that you drop your friends like a ton of bricks if they're having a hard time and need some support. Everyone, at times, will go through ups and downs in their life, and the help of friends can make those times a lot easier to deal with.

Be supportive, listen, help out when you can, and try to help them have more fun and laughter. Just being a listening ear at times can help, even if you're unable to do anything practical.

There are friends who are cheerful, upbeat, and fun to be around 90% of the time, who have odd crises in their lives that they need support for. There are other friends who seem to have crises, illnesses, dramas, upset, depression, hatred, anger, and negativity 90% of their lives, and are only cheerful now and then. These type of people may genuinely have tough lives… but others seem to thrive on the drama, and drag people down at the same time. Have you ever had one of those friends or acquaintances who seem to have problem after problem, but regardless of what 'solutions' you suggest they try, they seem to poo-poo the idea of help, which wears you out and leaves you thinking, 'Why did I bother?'

It's not easy to change your friendship group. Some of the techniques discussed later in this book are easier. But, you definitely do need to be aware of who you spend time with and try to surround yourself with people who will help you become the person you want to be. Ensure you spend time with people who have similar life goals to you, and who are supportive and encouraging.

The Bond of Friendship

Most humans have something in them that makes them want relationships with others. We live in a social world, where we take on board the standards, lifestyle, beliefs, philosophy, and habits of the people around us. Most of us tend to like others who share things in common with us.

If you have a lot of friends who are not keen on socialising and find it hard to make small talk, it isn't really surprising that you think similarly.

Consider, however, how it would be if you had lots of friends who loved nothing better than the excitement of talking to new people and finding out all about them.

Would you have a different approach to life? Would you change your views? Would you see people differently?

This is how my life started to change. In the past, I daren't speak in social situations, because I was terrified of what other people thought. I expected them to judge me (as I judged myself with an inner-critic). But, the more time I spent with people who were social, the more I realised that talking to people was easy, and people weren't something to be scared of.

I watched my friends who were bubbly and confident start conversations and I saw that others enjoyed being spoken to and engaged in conversation. Most people want to be recognized by others and made to feel like they matter and are special and different. People who are extroverts focus on the other person, rather than how they'll be viewed, and by doing this they find it easy to talk to others.

When you have lots of bubbly people around you, you will, without being aware of it, pick up on their behaviour and techniques.

Try to Find People You Admire

As mentioned previously, don't just cull everyone from your life who doesn't seem 'useful' to who you want to be as a person. I do believe that every single person is special and has a strength, ability, and/or personal characteristic that makes them uniquely valuable. You are able to help them find their strength.

But, you can make a concerted effort to be around people you admire, and who you would like to follow in the footsteps of. There are two key types: real-life mentors and aspirational mentors.

Real-life mentors are people you know in real life. These are people who you see have characteristics that you would like to have yourself. They could be a manager at work, a teacher at school or College, a leader in the community, or a friend or colleague.

If you can't think of anyone, don't worry too much about this at the moment. There will be lots of like-minded people you can connect with, and towards the end of this chapter, I'll share a technique for how you can find them immediately.

Aspirational mentors are people who you respect and would like to be like. These people can be dead or living. They can live or have lived anywhere in the world. These can be inspirational people who may be an entrepreneur, an artist, a musician, an athlete, a public speaker, a politician, an author, or anyone else. There are no restrictions to whom you can select.

It's perfectly possible to learn the secrets of success from people who have walked that walk before you. It can be a quicker way to learn. Tony Robbins, a great motivational speaker, talks about standing on the shoulders of giants for a metaphor that shows you can learn from people in the past. You don't have to go through their mistakes and failures, but skip over these and get to the direct results much quicker. By reading about successful people, you can feel like you know them well and they're sharing their knowledge and experience with you. By emulating their techniques and habits, you, too, can become successful. It's like a short-cut to success. My plan for this book is that I can pass on my knowledge to you, of how I overcame shyness, so that you can learn the tips and tricks it took me years to master, in just a few hours of reading the book.

Chapter 7

The Strength of a Smile

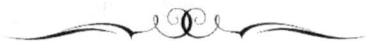

So, you've made it through the first half of the book! Well done! The first half of the book can be challenging because it's about examining yourself closely. We all put up quite a front - even to ourselves. It can be tough getting past that to see your true self. But, only when you have found out exactly where you're at, what changes you would like to make, and how you would like your future to be, can you move toward change.

In this chapter, there will be tips and techniques that you can apply to real-life to break out of your shell and become much less shy and more sociable. These aren't theoretical; they have been officially tried by myself and I know that they work. And they have worked for others, too. This means that should you choose to employ the techniques here, they will work for you too.

When you're reading through the book, you can view this as your training.

When you're not physically reading the book, it's a case of putting things into practice. You need to keep trying these techniques. Not every one that you try will go perfectly smoothly. But, stay open to the fact that you WILL become more sociable, and that every time you practice your techniques, you'll make progress and become less shy.

The key here is to make steady progress towards your goal; you don't have to be an expert in socialising from day one.

Let's get on with learning the first technique…

Smile like a Sunbeam

When I started University, I had a class that started at 8am on four of the weekdays.

Many students aren't really early-risers by choice, and I was no exception.

But, I was also right at the start of the process where I was determined to become less shy, and I came up with a great idea for my first week at college.

From my accommodation to the class, I would pass, on average, 20 people. On one of the mornings, I chose to smile at every single person I walked past.

I did wonder whether people would think I was crazy for grinning at them, or think I was mentally subnormal, or a weirdo.

But, whenever I thought about these worries, I would consider the book, *Control the Crazy*, that I had learned from. I would then re-think and find the next passing person who I could smile at.

I was surprised that almost 100% of the people I smiled at smiled back at me. It's kind of contagious. You know, like when you hear the sound of someone laughing, it makes you smile or laugh, too; smiling is the same. If someone smiles at you, you want to smile back. It also made me think that it didn't cost anything to smile, but by being friendly towards someone, I had made another person's day brighter for a little while.

I did this for a few weeks and then added in another layer. I decided to start saying, 'Good Morning' to everyone that I passed.

I was amazed at the response I received from people. You may think, 'Well of course people will respond positively.'

But this habit transformed my life, because when I reached my early morning University class, I would feel positive and uplifted. This enabled me to carry on being social in class, and I had the strength to answer questions from the teacher and join in discussions. It's a much better approach to be as smiley, cheerful, and upbeat to as many people as you can, than to keep your head down and ignore everyone you pass. If I'd ignored people en-route, I wouldn't have felt as enlivened, happy and sociable; and this may have meant that in class, I continued to myself, kept my head down, and did not join in with class discussion.

I had gotten over some of my fear of talking to others by starting with a simple smile. That's all it took; and you can change your life in the same way.

Research Supports Smiling

This may seem like a very basic technique, but I promise you it's a fantastic way to feel immediately ten times more confident.

Research from various studies will also support that smiling has enormous benefits, even if you smile when you're not in the mood. I figure that it's not possible to feel negative and positive simultaneously. You can cheer yourself up a lot if you decide to smile when you're feeling a bit down.

There's a book called *Smile: Secrets of the Healing Power of Your Smile*, where the author, Elan Sunstar, talks about how what you're feeling emotionally is influenced by your physical health and vice-versa. If you change one, the other changes too. When you smile at someone, this stops any negative feelings and you'll instead start to think of positive associations where you feel happy. By feeling positive emotionally, you'll be healthier physically, too. You can see the converse effect also; if you're feeling down, and very frowny, this can mean that you're more susceptible to picking up cold and stomach bugs and you can feel generally quite lethargic. Making yourself smile can really turn things around when you may not feel like it. Plaster a huge grin on your face; and I can guarantee you will start to feel better physically and emotionally.

When we feel positive inside, we feel more able to speak to others in a confident way.

I would assume that, mostly, you have negative associations and feel awkward when you think about talking to others. So, it's natural you'd avoid doing so, because we want to distance ourselves from anything that's uncomfortable and do what is comfortable instead. You may find it easier to keep quiet and safe from putting yourself into uncomfortable situations. But, you've always done this, and to be frank, it's not really worked well for you so far, has it? If it had been going so great, you wouldn't be feeling fed up. You wouldn't be feeling awkward or uncomfortable. You'd just roll with it and be having a great, anti-social time. You wouldn't have picked up this book about overcoming shyness. The very fact that you are reading this book suggests that you'd like to be able to talk to others, and you'd like to be less shy. There is a phrase, which I've used before in this book, but it's a great reminder when considering change, 'If you always do what you've always done, you will always get what you've always got.' You can't continue behaving in a certain way and expect a different outcome; it's just not going to happen.

But, remember earlier in the book when we spoke about creating a change? It's necessary for you to make that change within yourself. The fastest way to do this is by smiling at others, even if you have to fake a smile.

Become a Morning Person

I now love early mornings and the opportunity I

have to organize my thoughts during that time. I now wake up early, because it makes me feel good.

The part I dislike is that initial step out of a lovely, snuggly bed at 4am; but I can do this by training myself with a countdown from 3, which will be discussed later in Chapter 11.

I head immediately to the bathroom, and after brushing my teeth, head for a cold shower. Yes, cold!

I put a big smile on my face before the cold water hits me. I may look insane, but this motivates me. I gasp at the coldness, and it's the best feeling in the world. Cold water does have tremendous physical and mental health benefits; it'll do wonders for your circulatory system; it will make your skin glow and your hair shine; it will boost your immune system so you are less susceptible to colds and bugs; it will help to increase fertility, increase testosterone, and generally give you much more vitality and a sense of contentment. If you are a person who suffers from high blood pressure, then cold showers are not sensible, as they can make your blood vessels constrict. But, if you're otherwise healthy, you could try this and see how you feel. Cold water is great to wake you up and make you feel vitalized. Think of the difference too, when you're trying to work in a hot, stuffy room versus a cool room? When the room is too hot, you may start to either feel uncomfortable and sweat or else the heat can make you feel quite lethargic, drained, and devoid of all energy. It's not productive to be too warm. But, a cool room will keep you alert, focused and able to work. The cold water of the shower will make you really refreshed, alert, and able to think clearly.

In a similar manner to my physical morning shower, when I'm about to step into a social shower, where I may have felt a bit awkward and worried, I deliberately smile.

Smiling immediately reduces any anxiety. I can focus on what is happening around me instead of retreating to worrying thoughts in my mind; and I can focus on other people (rather than their opinion of me) and engage them in conversation.

You may consider forcing a smile a 'fake' way to live, and you may feel this would be a 'pretence' and a false, bizarre way to live. But, I promise you, after starting out with what may be a 'fake' smile for a few seconds, when you see real, genuine smiles returned to you, your smile will not be fake anymore; it'll spread and develop into a proper true grin. You'll make other people feel good by smiling; and this is a really positive thing.

Like Attracts Like

When you smile more at others and are more chatty with others, even in just a simplistic, greeting way, you will start attracting more positive people to you. People will start to want to talk with you. You won't have any concern over, 'What if I talk to someone and they don't speak back or think I'm odd, etc.?' People will make a beeline to speak with you and spend time with you. A happy person is a fun, positive, upbeat person to be around, and people are interested in happy people and what makes them behave that way.

Although, in the past, people talking to you may have worried you, you now do not have to worry about this. In Chapter 10 there will be some hints and tips for when people engage you in conversation and how to deal with it.

When you smile, people view you as an approachable, non-threatening, friendly person. Most people desire to protect themselves from being hurt or rejected. Without the need for you to even open your mouth to speak, smiling shows that you're a friendly person who does not want to hurt others. Let's face it – who would you rather approach? Someone who has their head down, shoulders slouched forward, who is not making eye contact, and is scowling? Or someone who is standing in an open, welcoming manner, whose eyes are bright and twinkling, and who has a lovely smile upon their face?

Prior to starting my smiling technique, often out of worry that someone would talk to me and I wouldn't know what to say, I would often hold my head low when I walked. I deliberately had a kind of blank expression on my face that gave nothing away. I was usually left alone by people; this appealed to me at the time, because for me, it was easier to be alone than to face my issues around socializing and risk being open and honest with others.

We can often make ourselves try to believe that we're happiest alone, not putting our thoughts or ideas out there and placing ourselves in a position of vulnerability. But, this isn't being truthful. When we connect with others, life is much more meaningful; it's much more fun when we smile at people and make connections. Memorable days in your life won't be the days where you successfully managed to avoid talking to anyone so they'll pass you by as unremarkable. Instead, they'll be the days you had an interesting conversation, threw some ideas around with someone, learned a new joke, learned a new recipe to try, perhaps made a new friend, or the first time you met your partner-to-be. All of these memorable days are based upon interactions and connections with others.

Smile Training

You do need to smile a lot every day. It's as important to keep practicing your smile as it would be to practice running if you were attempting a marathon. You can smile at any time around your house, initially, without having to smile at another physical person.

You can practice smiling when you take a shower, whilst you're hoovering, when you make a cup of tea, or when you cut the lawns. Smile at your pets. Start out by smiling around the house.

Try to use as many of your facial muscles when you smile as possible. Don't do this half-heartedly; really throw yourself into smiling, and use all your muscles to make a massive smile that wrinkles your eye lines, too.

If you live in the house with another person, whether it's your partner, parents, family, or room-mates, they may initially think you've gone a bit mad. Don't worry about them; instead lend them this book, and especially encourage them to read this chapter so they have a better understanding of what is going on. If they can understand and support you better, and even learn a few tips and tricks for themselves to apply, then it's all for the better.

When you're ready, you need to then be practicing these smiles out in public. There will be lots of opportunities for you to do this: when you go to fetch a newspaper or pint of milk; when you put the rubbish outside; standing at a bus or train stop, and so on. Next, extend this smile to your work or school/college colleagues, with staff in shops, or at restaurants. With time, you will become known as the smiley person, the person who is always cheerful, always positive, and happy. And people love enthusiastic, happy people because they're a pleasure to be around. Happiness is contagious. It's motivating, inspiring, and will automatically make you appear a more confident person. A happy person appears in control, less stressed, with less issues and dramas.

It is perfectly natural that you may feel a bit out of your depth and uncomfortable at first. But, I can guarantee that other people aren't spending as much time thinking about you, or making judgements and critical comments about you, as you believe. People have better things to be doing; they're getting on with living their own lives and dealing with their own issues. This was another liberating moment for me, when I realized this. You need to believe this, too. Don't concern yourself with other people's opinions. Simply mind your own business, do everything in your own life to the best of your ability, and let other people worry about their lives, thoughts, and opinions.

If ever you start to worry about smiling and thinking you look silly, stop and thank your mind for its concerns. Then allow yourself to smile a big, massive grin once again! This can actually be quite a good technique for dealing with 'well intended' advice throughout life, too. If ever you feel someone is giving you advice that you didn't actually ask for or says things like "I tell you what you should do ..." even if you think their advice is ridiculous, rather than get into an argument with them about it, you can thank them for their concerns, smile, and do your own thing! My Mum gave me that advice for what people will suggest when it comes to looking after/raising children, because everyone thinks they're the expert and knows best. So, just thank them, smile and nod, and go ahead and do things your own way. It's good advice for dealing with others, as well as your own negative thoughts.

Chapter 8

Nonverbal Cues

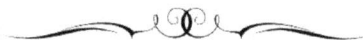

N onverbal cues are also known as body language. It's a key way we communicate with others, whether we're aware of it or not. It is said that 55% of what we communicate is through our body language, 38% through the tone of what we have to say, and just 7% of what we communicate is via the words.

So, if you worry greatly about speaking in front of other people and hope that you don't trip over your words or say the wrong thing, these statistics should take away a lot of your worry. The key thing you should be focusing on is your nonverbal cues.

There is a fabulous technique that I'll share with you; and it's easy to apply in social situations. When you do this, and adjust your nonverbal cues in this way, you will look and feel confident.

Ok, so here it is …

A-E of Confidence

By following these techniques, you will immediately be much more confident and animated in your stance and your conversation. It's a great hint for when you're meeting someone for the first time, speaking with a group of people, talking to your manager, or anywhere else. You need to recall A-E:

A: Adjust your body so that your shoulders are up and back - and stand firm.

B: Breathe deeply in through your nose and out through your mouth.

C: Clasp your hands together; this gives you something practical to do with them, so that you don't feel they're hanging there awkwardly. You won't be tempted to tap or fidget, and you'll look poised and in control.

D: Display your smile – place a big grin on your face.

E: Eye contact – ensure you look at people directly.

A-E has helped me so much in social situations that I didn't initially feel comfortable in. If ever I feel nervous, feel my hands starting to sweat, and begin to feel jittery, I remind myself of A-E and it helps to calm me down - and make me look much more confident.

Each of the A-E steps, only take a few seconds to achieve. I will now talk in a bit more detail about each of them:

Adjust Your Shoulders

When your shoulders stoop or slouch forward, this makes you look shy, indecisive, and can give a lazy appearance. It can make you look a bit shifty, too.

People will sometimes refer to it as 'slouching.' People may assume that if you slouch, you're lazy, because they'll think if you can't be bothered to stand correctly with good posture, your other habits connected with work and life will be sloppy, half-hearted, and lazy too. This may be grossly unfair and untrue, but for people meeting you for the first time, or who do not know you well, this is the first impression they'll get of you. First impressions can shape how people perceive you in the future. They'll look for behaviour that reinforces their impression.

Now, whilst you may be the most honest, hard-working person in the world, your body language may send off different signals. There's an easy solution. Stand up straight, push your shoulders back and feel like you're having a good stretch of your rib cage. This will give you much more poise and will make you appear smart, confident, and like a go- getter.

I'll be perfectly honest and say that I find this habit hard to adhere to. My partner often reminds me to stand tall and not slouch. Whilst I found this a tad annoying at first, I know that my partner I right to point this out; and the reminders help me to focus on this and become better at it. If you would benefit from adjusting your posture, you could enlist the help of your partner, a family member, or a work colleague to mention it to you whenever they see that you're slouching. It will definitely help you down the line.

Not to mention the fact that having better posture

has enormous health benefits, anyhow. Posture, i.e., the way that you hold and position yourself, not only makes you look confident and better, it has lots of key health benefits too. Having good posture can prevent you from developing pain in your back, neck, and shoulders. Good posture can prevent injuries and other health issues. Whilst spines have some curvature naturally, when you slouch, you're adding much more unhealthy curvature. You can cause your body to become misaligned. People often spend a lot of time and money with practitioners, having their body gently realigned. If you keep on slouching this can damage your spine and make it more likely to succumb to injuries. When your spine does not have good alignment, this places pressure on other joints, such as hips and knees. Your balance may be affected; you won't digest your food as easily; and you won't breathe as easily.

You can be aware of your posture, not only when you're standing up, but when you're sitting too. Ensure you keep most of your weight on the balls of your feet when you're standing, and aim to keep your head upright and level.

There is also something known as the Alexander Technique which could be well worth researching and investigating. Many celebrities and leaders follow this technique. It is all about finding balance, poise, good posture, and coordination, which runs through all you do in life. Having good posture can help you develop personally; it makes you more self-aware and mindful, and it will help you to more easily learn new skills and habits to transform your life. Practicing the Alexander Technique can prevent pain, injury, tension, and stiffness so that you move gracefully and with poise. It will give you the confidence to deal with everyday life stresses where you may previously have tensed due to nerves - for example, when speaking to someone on the phone or in person, having a meeting, or giving a presentation, etc. You'll learn techniques wherein you can identify stress and how to prevent yourself from reacting to these instances. Once you've learned the technique, it's yours to use for the rest of your life. You'll learn to have balance in your mind and body. It will give you more stamina; you'll learn how to relax; and you will have great clarity of thought. Singers and actors often learn this method because it can also help with breathing and vocal problems, too, making it great to help performers in music, drama and sports. It can also help people with their presentation skills and make you more eloquent. The technique can help throughout pregnancy and will generally improve your balance and coordination.

Breathe Deeply

Having a good posture and stance, with your shoulders back and a wide-open chest, will help with your breathing. Take a deep breath in through your nose; ensure you count to five before exhaling the breath through your mouth slowly (in a controlled way, not in an explosion of breath). As you're breathing out, imagine that all the stress, angst, anxiety, and concern you have in your body and mind is being breathed out of your body too.

Another way of getting rid of any anxiety, negative thoughts, and clutter that's in your head when you feel your head is too busy with thoughts, can be to imagine someone holding up an ice cube to your forehead. Imagine the coldness from the ice cube dissipating backwards as the ice melts, and trickling through your mind towards the back of your head, clearing out any of those hot, angry thoughts and replacing them with coolness and calmness. It's a nice visualisation technique that has helped me on many occasions.

If you are tense and coiled like a spring, this will show in your body language and the person you're speaking with, even if only subconsciously, will feel that you're uncomfortable. It can change your interaction entirely.

If you take two of the deep breaths discussed above, and perhaps apply the ice-cube technique to clear your mind, you will feel much calmer and more grounded and able to focus on people and what they have to say - rather than panicked and stressed.

Clasp Hands Together

Sometimes in a social situation, it feels as though my arms grow as long as the Mr. Men character, Mr. Tickle's, and I don't know where to place my arms or hands. I almost feel like I have as many arms as an octopus - and they get in the way! Having a stance where you position your hands makes you less self-conscious of them. You then won't fidget, put them in your pockets, pick at threads on your sleeves, tap your fingers, or twiddle your thumbs. It gives your hands a purpose.

If you're prone to twirling your hair or fiddling with your collar, or a ring or bracelet, once again these fidgety non-verbal cues will make anyone you're talking to subconsciously aware that you're feeling awkward. It may rub off on them and they can begin to feel a bit awkward, too.

There are some places where it's suitable to hold your hands. As a general guide, it can be advisable to have your hands near your chest when you talk and in your lap when you listen to others.

There are different types of ways that you can clasp your hands. You can have your fingers clasped flat to your hand or have them with finger-tips touching in a steeple position (which I personally think gives a calmer persona). But, the stance needs to be one that you feel comfortable with. You can practice this at home, in front of a full-body mirror, to see what you prefer the look of before trying it in public.

Display Your Smile

You've had plenty of practice smiling now, right? You need to keep smiling when you're talking with others. Make yourself smile and nod in the right places, too. This shows that you're friendly and open to their ideas. It shows you're listening to them and actively interacting with what they have to say. When you smile, it serves a dual purpose of giving you confidence and giving a boost of positivity to the other person, who will then respond to you well, too. If you don't smile and nod, the other person will feel quite disarmed and may worry that they're boring you or that you don't really want to be speaking to them. They may wrap the conversation up much quicker than they would normally have done.

Eye Contact

If you struggle to look people in the eyes, there's a way of looking like you are whilst not actually doing so. I'll explain this technique more in just a few moments. When you're in a conversation with someone, looking them in the eyes shows you're interested in them. They trust you and feel happy to talk to you. If eye-to-eye contact makes you feel a little uncomfortable, then try instead starting off looking at the person's nose, mouth, or the space in between their eyebrows until you feel better about looking them in the eye. This is great, because it's still around about the right place on their face. If you feel uncomfortable with direct eye contact at any point throughout the conversation, have a break and look at their nose instead.

So, you've mastered smiling and having a wonderful stance and calming, approachable body language. You're in a good place to try this out with people.

Chapter 9

The Metre Rule

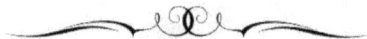

Y ou are over half way to becoming super confident by having discovered how to control your body language. What we'll now focus on is actually speaking with people.

Over the years, you'll have become good at putting yourself in the background and away from situations where you have to speak with others. But, I 100% promise you, I've got some great news. It is MUCH easier to speak with people than what you've been worrying about. Once you start to do it, you will wonder why you've not done it much sooner. You will wonder what the big deal was. I'm not trivialising how you feel when you're shy, because believe me, I've had a lifetime of it. But, just when you cease to be and decide to change, life feels like you're really alive and living properly for the first time.

With just a few simple techniques, you'll be able to speak with anyone, from any walk of life, and engage them in interesting conversation. Sometimes we may worry that we're not of the same educational status or perhaps same class/social background as another person. This can make us hesitant to engage them in conversation, in case they think us foolish. Firstly, people who have been brought up well will have the manners to converse with you about most things. If there's ever anything you don't understand in a conversation, be brave enough to acknowledge this and ask the other person to explain. People generally like to teach others new things and to help them learn and understand. No-one will ever think you foolish for wanting to learn, because people love to teach and demonstrate their knowledge. My advice would be to never pretend you're knowledgeable on a subject that you're not; stick to what you know and can confidently talk about. And anything you don't know, take as an opportunity to learn about and ask questions. We'll cover more about the power of questions in Chapter 10.

A metre is 100 cm (or just over 3 foot). You need to pretend that you carry an invisible ruler or tape-measure of this length around with you. If anyone steps into this metre zone, you need to try to have a conversation with them. This is the new rule that you need to follow. Whilst you may be hesitant at first, I promise with time, you'll actually go out of your way to walk closer to people to get them to fall within your metre zone.

If you're a shy person, and have gone through life avoiding people deliberately, I know this may be initially terrifying to you. It's OK to be scared. But, please keep yourself open to change and to trying this out.

It is really easy to do.

Talk to Strangers

As children we're given the opposite advice of 'Don't talk to strangers' - and this is sensible advice for children to heed. But, when you reach the adult world, you need to talk to every person you get the chance to.

When you talk to as many people as possible, you open up the possibility that these people 'could' become good friends. You may find out that you have certain things in common with them, enjoy chatting with them, and want to spend more time with them. If you don't talk to people, it can make things at the workplace really tough, relationships non-existent, and you can become unhappy. Shyness really can impact you negatively. I know from experience. I once had a VERY small circle of friends - to the extent I had one real best friend and no partner for years. The people I spent a lot of my time with were my parents. And, whilst it's nice that we're a close family, there are certain activities that it's just much better to do with a group of friends instead, such as going to the cinema, going to parties, and fun days out. Certain things are more fun to do with people of a similar age to yours, without a generation gap. You need to chat with others to learn more about them and to make informed decisions about who you'd like to spend more time with and have as friends.

As human beings, we need to have meaningful

connections with people. It can be a lonely, depressing life if you don't have friends. It's nice to have people you can call up and chat with on the phone. It's nice to have people you can go out for day trips with, share meals with, go to the cinema with, have cups of tea and cake with, play a round of golf with, watch a football game with, and so on. I want to assist you to be able to communicate with ease and express yourself.

What Will I Say?

Part of what stops us talking to strangers is our worry that they may think we're foolish. Or, we worry that they may not find us interesting. Or, we don't want to take up their time. We worry about what is the right or wrong thing to say.

There will be times in your life when you've wanted to speak with a person, but then you've become all flustered and can't think of a single sensible, coherent sentence to say to them. I've done this numerous times in the past when, due to nerves, my mind has gone so completely blank that I can't think of a single thing to say. I was once asked, "What music do you like?" and I couldn't think of a single band/group/singer. It was frustrating and ridiculous – I love music, but I couldn't even remember what CDs I had in the house or what I listened to on Spotify.

There's a great technique that will start you off with the Metre Rule; it's like a magic spell.

The Magic Spell

The magic spell is four special words, an incantation that you need to say out loud: "Hello, how are you?"

You're probably thinking to yourself, 'Is that all there is to it? Surely that won't work!!!!'

But, I promise you faithfully - and scientific research supports it - that this simple technique works!!!! So, this is perfect if you have concerns about what to say to start a conversation.

This technique above was learned by Vanessa Van Edwards, who I saw speak at a conference in Nashville. She studies people and their behaviour by profession; it's her area of expertise.

She has said that people wrack their brains for something which is unusual or funny to say, or something to try and make them look clever. But this line is 100% effective to start a conversation. It doesn't need to be any more complex than that. By keeping it simple, your comment isn't going to unnerve the other person, either. It's a relatively easy question that they'll be able to respond to.

So, if you say that line to anyone who is within a metre distance of you, you will soon start to have a lot of conversations. There are other techniques you can do when you're meeting people after that line which are also effective:

Shake Hands with Them

This isn't just to be professional or formal; there is a scientific explanation too. When you shake hands with someone, because your hands touch, you'll release oxytocin in your bodies, and this will forge a closer connection between the two of you. The other person will trust you more; it will form a bond. When we shake someone's hand, subconsciously we are working out whether we can trust them. If we believe we can, the brain releases oxytocin that tells us it is safe to trust them. At the same time as oxytocin, dopamine will be released, and this is like our reward and pleasure. Oxytocin makes us trust and become more generous, increases empathy, and will make us more understanding to others and allow us to see other people's perspectives.

This book won't go into the details connected to handshakes, though you could do further research on the Internet about this. But, ensure your hands are dry, have a firm grip that isn't too weak and floppy like a dead fish and also isn't overly aggressive. When you're shaking hands with someone, you're not trying to prove how strong you are. If the other person seems to be squeezing tightly as a show of strength, let them; it's obviously important to them for some reason.

Introductions

Try to keep your introduction brief, short, and sweet - and remember that you want to learn about the person you're speaking to. Here are some examples:

If you were at a gym you could say, "Hello, how

are you? I'm XXX. What type of workout are you planning today?"

If you were in a coffee shop you could say, "Hello, how are you? I'm XXX. Do you have a particular coffee you would recommend?"

Once they reply, you can drive the conversation with more questions. There is a chapter, later in this book, which shows how powerful questions can be.

You'll be able to judge the best time in the conversation to shake their hand and make your introductions. Don't worry about saying the right words and remember that's actually a very small part (7%) of the whole communication. Follow the process as set out here.

Top Tip: It's much better to start a conversation than worry too much about trying to say the perfect thing.

One you've made your introduction and have got the conversation started, there are other hints and tips to keep that conversation going nicely.

Keep Smiling - and Nod, Too

If you're a person who is trying to be less shy, smiling and nodding will be your best friends. We can worry a lot before starting to speak with someone, as we think we need to control the conversation and have the right thing to say. Don't worry about this; just let it flow. If you're constantly trying to steer the conversation or planning what you'll say next, you're not truly listening and paying attention to what is said. Just ease into the conversation and you'll find it'll be much more natural and easy going. It's perfectly natural to have pauses in conversation and it is good to allow the other person to think and digest what has been said. Don't feel the need to fill every gap with babble.

When I speak with someone, I try to have an 80/20 rule, where I will get the other individual talking to me 80% of the time whilst I, myself, talk the remaining 20%.

This is because a lot of people like to talk about themselves. It makes them feel valued and appreciated, and like they're interesting and have knowledge to pass on that is useful to others, interesting, or amusing. I'm not just doing this to flatter their ego and butter them up; I genuinely believe this to be true, too. I think every single person has interesting things that they can share with you. When you're talking to someone new, you won't always want to open up and share your deepest thoughts immediately; but when you are comfortable in someone's company, it's much easier to discuss what you're thinking.

So, we need to make the person feel as comfortable as possible so that they're relaxed and at ease. Whilst the other person is talking, if you smile and nod, this will encourage them to keep talking. If you're a good listener, this will make you just as popular as a being good speaker - because people do love people who will listen to them and let them talk and throw ideas around.

If you apply your listening skills whenever you're in a social setting, you will be part of amazing conversations.

Ending the Conversation

When the conversation seems to be coming to its natural end, it's a good technique to enquire about the other person's future. This isn't intended to be really deep and meaningful (and not something like, "And where do you see yourself in five years' time?" That's more of an interview question), but simply something along the lines of:

"Do you have any plans for this afternoon?"

"Are you doing anything nice this weekend?"

This will allow your conversation to have a smooth finish, so that when you shake hands with them and say goodbye, you can add a personal touch of:

"It was lovely to speak with you, XXX. I hope you and your family have an excellent time this weekend at the Hockey game!"

Ending a conversation well is just as important as your initial impression. Taking the time to inquire about their plans, remembering their name, and making your conversation-end personal shows that you really care about them and were interested in what they had to say. You'll both end the conversation feeling good.

If you're chatting with someone and the conversation ends more sharply than you'd hoped for, don't worry or stress about it. There could be a million and one reasons why this has happened. It could be that they want to talk to others in the room; they may have a meeting at a certain time; they could need to use the toilet. Always keep smiling and, if you get the chance, let them know that you enjoyed the conversation.

If the person you've been chatting with seems like someone you'd like to keep in touch with, then a good strategy can be to ask if they're on Facebook. Lots of people are on Facebook or on LinkedIn, and it's a bit less personal than calling or texting a person. Especially if the person is the opposite sex to you, it can come across as a bit less like you're asking for a phone number for a date. If they are on Facebook or LinkedIn and do want to connect, it can be nice to pass someone your phone and let them put their own name in; it again lets the person trust you. For most people their phone is important to them, because it contains their contacts, photos, etc. Handing someone your phone shows that you are choosing to trust them.

If someone doesn't have Facebook or LinkedIn, or if they don't want to stay connected, don't be upset or take it personally. It won't happen often, but you can still be grateful for the conversation you've had; it's given you the chance to be confident and get some good conversational practice in.

Now, you've had a go at using the Metre Rule. You don't need to do this EVERY time that someone is within a metre of you; but please try to do it at least once a day. You'll be doing really well if you've started the conversation off and should feel very proud of yourself.

Chapter 10

Asking Effective Questions

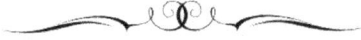

———————— ⟨◎⟩ ————————

This is a key take-away from this book. If you only remember one thing from the book, please remember this: If you're wanting to try to keep the other person in a conversation talking for 80% of the time, so that you're able to listen and interact with them and be perceived as a person who is fun to have a conversation with, then you need to ask that person questions!

When I learned this tip, it truly did make a big change to my life. I carefully considered what it was that scared me about talking to people.

I figured out that for me, I was a bit scared of people - and I wasn't sure how to remain calm and avoid getting flustered in a conversational situation. But, when I asked the other person a heap of questions, this worked a treat. Asking questions allows you to deflect attention and the conversation away from yourself, onto them.

When you ask another person questions, you'll learn much more about them, as well as about a wide variety of topics. You'll learn about yourself, too. It's important to ask questions in a non-interrogation type way though; you don't want to bark questions at them aggressively in a rapid fire. It is better to use gentle, probing questions to show that you're interested and would like to find out more and to prolong the conversation.

When you ask a person questions, it's nice to try and find something that you both can relate to and have in common. If you feel shy and awkward, it can be because you think you're the only person who feels like this.

But, here's something to think about. All human beings do share a common trait. We all want to be accepted and loved, and we all have certain things we're afraid of. If you take the time to connect with a person and find out more about them, you'll discover that they probably have one of these areas of their life that they aren't as happy with as they could be. You are capable of connecting with anyone. I believe that every, single person has something interesting to share and talk about. Your mission, should you choose to accept it, is to find what their interest is, find something that connects the two of you, and try to expand this connection.

Questions are Powerful

In the past, I worked at a coffee shop. The mornings were often frantic, with people popping in to purchase teas and coffees for their morning commute to work. Regardless of how busy each morning was, I tried to ask each customer a question or pay each customer a compliment that would improve their day. This was a great technique to come across as friendly and interested, as well as offer good, personal customer service, getting to know my customers better and helping them to feel welcome and appreciated in the shop

One day, a gentleman in his thirties came in for his coffee with his children, who were boisterously running about. He looked very tired, probably due to caring for his children. As I passed him his coffee, I asked him, "What do you like best about being a Dad?" He hadn't been expecting the question and seemed initially a bit thrown by it. But after a few moments he replied, "Their love, which is unconditional. You just can't describe it."

He smiled and walked away after placing a tip in the jar. When answering the question, his face was filled with joy. The tip he left was very kind and appreciated. This exchange taught me something important - that when we ask another person the correct question, we can change their day. We can make them feel grateful for life even if they'd been having a momentary blip; they can feel noticed appreciated, and valued. My question to him probably took him away from how hectic the day was, how boisterous his children were being, and all the worries about the school run and issues that lay ahead for him at work that day - and instead reminded him about what was truly important to him and what he was doing it all for.

What Should I Ask?

How well you know a person will determine the level that a question should be pitched at. If you're meeting someone for the first time, you may not want to dive in with a really deep, meaningful question such as, "What's the meaning of life?" Conversely, if you've been dating someone for a number of years, you don't want to be finding out "What do you enjoy doing in your spare time?"

When you're just getting to know someone, here are some questions you could ask:

What are your interests?

How would you describe your family?

Do you have a favourite figure from history?

What's your background?

What do you enjoy most about being a parent?

If you were hosting a dinner party and could invite anyone from the past or present, who would you invite, and why?

If anything was possible with no constraints, how would you choose to spend your day?

Where in the world would you like to visit? Why?

Is there a book that changed your outlook on life?

These questions go beyond general introductory chit-chat and allow you to learn more about a person and who they really are, without making them feel awkward.

If you feel these questions are still too intense for you, there are some simpler ones here:

Are you employed? How do you spend your time?

Where did you study?

Where did you spend your childhood?

Do you have a favourite restaurant?

What's your favourite film?

Tell me about your best friend.

Where's the nicest holiday you've ever been on?

You don't have to worry about your exact words; what is far more crucial is that you're talking to a person - and you're asking questions that will get them thinking, talking, and engaging with you.

When someone replies to your questions, this sometimes leaves room to think of other questions that spring from the information they've told you. So, keep on questioning, listening, and commenting about their information. You can always have some standby questions at hand if you're worried about gaps in the conversation. But do listen actively and carefully, too. Don't worry about having to fill every gap or pause. Let the conversation take its natural course.

Actively Listen

Often when we're in a conversation, we can be focused upon trying to get our own points in or working out what our next comment or question will be. But, when we're doing this, we're not truly listening to the other person with our full attention. If you're a person who does this, really firmly work on damping down all the thoughts in your mind whilst you listen and concentrating on the other person and what they have to say. If you're busy thinking of what to say next, there can sometimes be a tendency to jump in and interrupt before the other person has finished speaking, which can come across as a little rude.

There are 5 things you can do in order to actively listen:

1. Give positive feedback to the person. You can do this in 2 ways - verbal and nonverbal. Verbal would include little affirmations such as, "Yes," "I agree," or, "I understand." Nonverbal feedback can include looking at them, nodding, and smiling.

2. Clarify any misunderstandings. If you don't totally understand what someone means when they're talking to you, you can ask them questions like, "Could you explain that?" When you ask questions like that, ensure it's clear that you're wanting to understand better and that you're not challenging them in an aggressive or sarcastic way. People don't mind explaining things; they want you to understand what they mean.

3. It can be a good idea to repeat back to the person what they've told you, but in your own words and phrasing. This allows them to see if you've understood what they're saying. You can start your comments with phrases such as, "If I've understood your meaning, you're stating that ...." And then you can end with, "Is that correct?"

4. Don't interrupt the person as mentioned above; otherwise it can seem like you're rude, in a hurry for them to get to the point, or that you think you know better than them what they want to say. Other than making verbal feedback noises, or asking a question if you're unsure what is meant, try to listen in silence until the other person has finished speaking – even if this goes on for a while. Be patient, listen carefully, and drink in what they're saying. When you reply to them, try to ignore any heated emotions or emotional argument which can be used to sway you, and instead focus on logical, hard facts. By doing this, you're responding rather than emotionally reacting, which can often be quite knee-jerk. When you're emotional, you can often give a heated response, which you later regret when you've calmed down and have thought things through.

5. Be open, non-judgemental, patient, and neutral in your responses. When you're listening to someone, the key thing is that you understand what they want to say, not whether you agree or

disagree with them. When you keep yourself open, you'll be able to hear more of what they really mean and what they believe to be true. After this, you can talk about ideas.

The more you practice listening to people, the more you'll begin to hear the emotion in their words. This tells you much more than the words on their own.

Also look closely at what the person's nonverbal cues are. If the emotion in their voice doesn't seem to tally up with the words they are saying, then look at their body language, too.

If you've ever seen the TV show *Lie to Me* with the actor, Tim Roth, it's a brilliant programme that looks at micro-expressions and body language to determine people's guilt or non-involvement in crimes. Micro-expressions are about reading a person's face. Micro-expressions only stay on a person's face for a fraction of the time; they can pull a fake smile or create fake tears after this. You have to look quickly to see the micro-expression; it's involuntary and they can't help but do it. This could perhaps be the fraction of a smirk if someone is secretly pleased about something, even though they're pretending they're not. It could be the fraction of a frown if they were really hurt about something. In the programme *Lie to Me*, people would often be videoed - and it's only when the film was slowed right down in slow-motion that you could see the micro-expression. You can develop your skills in body language, following the tips in this book and using your powers of observation. There are seven key micro-expressions. These include surprise, fear, disgust, anger, happiness, sadness, and contempt/hate.

With body language, which is a bit more noticeable than micro-expressions, you can most likely tell those same seven categories by looking at someone's face, unless they're very adept at lying or acting. With other body language knowledge, you can look at someone's eyes. If someone's eyes are very dilated, this can be a sign of attraction or desire. If someone blinks a lot, they can be nervous, and this can be a sign of them feeling a bit agitated or distressed and uncomfortable. Or, you can look at someone's lips. If they bite their lips, this could be a sign they're worried. If they purse their lips tightly together, this can be a sign that they've found something distasteful or disapprove of something. If someone covers their mouth with their hand, this could be to hide an expression, such as a smile or a frown.

It's possible for people to make various gestures and signals with their hands when they talk. Do be VERY careful to research hand-gestures, though, if you're in an international crowd and talking, because some hand gestures which seem innocuous to you could, in other parts of the world, have an offensive meaning. You could upset people without realizing. Gestures can be hard to interpret and the context does indeed need to be fully taken into account. For example, a clenched fist can at times represent anger and at other times can be used as a symbol for solidarity. Having a thumbs up or thumbs down can show that you either agree and approve or disagree and disapprove. The finger and thumb touching to make an O shape can mean 'OK' in some cultures. In others, it's offensive and means that you think the person is nothing. In yet other cultures, it's quite vulgar; so do be very careful who you use this around - or avoid it completely unless just with friends. Having two fingers in a V shape, can celebrate a victory or can be used to symbolize a swear word/gesture – again, use this with caution.

You can als0 analyse body language by looking at someone's arms. If they're crossed in front of them, this can show they're putting a barrier between you and them; it's quite a defensive gesture. It shows that they may be closed to anything you have to say to them because of this barrier. If someone puts their hands on their hips, this can be a symbol of being in control and may show some aggression. If someone is rapidly tapping their fingers, this could indicate impatience, boredom, or frustration because it's an outwards display of being a bit agitated and quite fidgety. You can also look at legs; if someone has their legs crossed, you can get an impression of how favourably they're viewing you based on whether they are crossed in your direction or away from you. It's typically more favourable if they're crossed towards you rather than away from you.

We've spoken a little about posture already, but

how someone sits, whether they're keeping their body compact and tight, hiding their body with their limbs, or they have a more open posture, can let you know whether they're a bit unfriendly and anxious (closed) or friendly and open (open posture).

When you're speaking with someone new, be sure not to invade their personal space; leave a suitable distance between you and them. As a general rule, about 1.5 to 4 feet away is acceptable. You can judge how comfortable the other person feels as you're talking to them. If they step back a little, it's clear they need a little bit more space between you. If they step forward slightly, they're interested in getting to know you better. Some cultures differ in how they perceive personal space, with some cultures being happier standing very close to one another and others preferring more distance.

When you're next out and about, ensure that you speak to at least one person. Take on board where you are, try to find some common ground between you, and start talking to them.

It's perfectly fine if the conversation is brief and doesn't extend too much. This is about you having the confidence to speak with others and being brave enough to do something about it. Having been a very shy person myself, I can absolutely promise you that when you pluck up the courage and start doing this, firstly you'll see that people aren't that scary to talk to. Most people are courteous and friendly and only too happy to talk. But, once you've chatted, even if it wasn't the most ground-breaking conversation ever, you'll feel very proud of yourself for having initiated the chat.

Chapter 11

The Secret Recipe

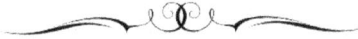

Y ou may have previously heard about some of the techniques in this book. It can be useful to have a reminder sometimes to make the idea seem worthwhile. Other times, we need the idea put to us in just a slightly different way that makes it make sense to us.

In this book, I've given you hints and tips that have been used by thousands of people over the years, which have helped them to become less shy and express themselves with more ease.

This last technique, however, you may never have heard of previously - and this is the secret recipe you need to bring all of this together and make it work.

You may in the past have known how to do something, or what you should be doing, but haven't done it. (Think of diets/exercise regimes for instance – it's not rocket-science, but is much harder to do).

How many times in the past have you thought about what you 'could' be saying to someone who looked like an interesting person, but instead you remained quiet and reserved and didn't speak?

The moments where you prevent yourself from doing things end right now.

Stop Sabotaging Yourself

You may find a lot of helpful videos on YouTube that could be immensely useful to give you information or change your approach to life. In one video called 'How to Stop Screwing Yourself Over' by Mel Robbins, she emphasizes that we already know what we want. But, when we're thinking about acting on something, our emotions and thoughts battle with one another - and it's our emotions that win. It's hard to talk yourself into an action, no matter how logical it may seem, when you're scared.

So, for example, you may have battled with thoughts such as:

'They look like a nice group of people over there who I'd like to sit with and chat, but I daren't go and speak with them.'

Or, 'I have some ideas I'd like to share with people at work, but I don't have the confidence to speak out.'

Or, 'I'd like to ask that person on a date to the cinema, but what if they say no?'

Emotions and feelings can be important, and they can work well for us or work against us, depending on whether they make us act, or we fail to act because of them.

So, you may know what to do; and you have your

motivation for why you want to do it. But, that isn't always enough to spur you on to action. There is, however, a solution.

In the video mentioned above by Mel Robbins, if you want to act on an aim, you MUST do this within 5 seconds, or else your emotions will take over and will stop you acting.

What you can do to force yourself to move is start a 5 second countdown. So, for example, if you'd just been to a gig of a musician you liked and, after the show, they were mingling among the crowds chatting to people, when you see them, you have...

5... 4... 3... 2... 1... to say "Hello. How are you? My name is X."

If you're in a workplace meeting and your manager asks, "Does anyone have anything to add about how we could tackle the X issue....?" you have...

5... 4... 3... 2... 1... to start speaking up and sharing your ideas.

There will be lots of opportunities in a day where you can apply this rule to force yourself to act, become less shy, and start expressing your thoughts.

Ralph Emerson speaks about how people who act are powerful; whilst those who do not move and do something are powerless.

So, you need to stop analysing and dwelling over

every aspect of your life and just do things, live life, and act exactly how you want to. You start to become powerful when you make the effort to just do things.

You could spend years of your life, or indeed your whole life, just reading self-help books, listening to podcasts, watching seminars... and still nothing much has changed in your life, until you make the decision to change and act. You need to be courageous and take that first step. If you just keep waiting until the perfect moment, you'll keep waiting forever.

So, this secret recipe can change your life, because it's all about you physically acting very quickly - within 5 seconds.

Twist to the Recipe

When I tried the 5 Second Rule strategy of knowing I wanted to act, just counting down 5 seconds, and ensuring I had acted within this time, I got brilliant results immediately.

I managed to keep getting up at 4am and jumping into a cold shower. I countdown to get in the shower.

If I was out and about at the shops and wanted to ask someone I'd not met before a question or pay someone a compliment, I would start the 5 second countdown.

If I'd been putting off making a telephone call at work, I would start the countdown.

But, I did make a small tweak and twist to the

recipe.

I felt that counting down 5 seconds was a bit too long. It was long enough for my brain to start going into a panic - and I'd have time to start talking myself out of things. So, I cut down my countdown to 3 seconds and this worked much better for me.

I'm not perfect every single time with any of the techniques I've suggested in the book. I do still feel afraid from time to time, and occasionally I won't speak to someone when I wish I would. But, if these instances occur, I don't let it stress me out too much, and I don't dwell on it and think about it for ages. Because becoming less shy is something which I've committed to work at for life, and I'll gradually keep on improving.

So let's try out the exercise right now. You need to think of something that you've been procrastinating about. What is something that you've had on a 'to do' list but still haven't actually got around to doing? It could be that you keep saying to a friend, "We must catch up for coffee," but then you don't. Or you could owe someone an apology that you haven't given them yet. Or, there could be part of your house that you've been meaning to sort out, such as a drawer, a cupboard, or a room.

Once you've focused on what it is that you should have done, put down this book and start your countdown, whether that is from 5, or 3, whatever works best for you, to get you to act:

3... 2... 1...

If you start to think of all the excuses under the sun for why you shouldn't do this, put those out of your mind and start your timer once again. Don't waste another minute of your life; just get things done. When you're next in a social situation, try this technique as often as you can.

Using this technique will allow you to achieve immediate results and start having meaningful conversations with others. It's a call to action which has an immediate result. It stops you procrastinating, stops you putting things off until 'someday' – because you need to act now to change your life for the better.

Chapter 12

Lifelong Learning and Development

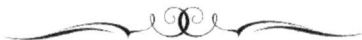

Have you tried the 5 or 3 Second Rule? How did you get on? What are your thoughts and feelings about it?

If you haven't yet, then again, put down this book and do it right away!

This book is meant to encourage you to make changes and act - so that you can become more of who you truly are.

Assuming you have made some of these changes and used some of the other hints and tips within this book, we can move on. This book is coming to an end shortly.

There is No End

When I read *Control the Crazy* for the very first time, it changed my life. I have since gone back and read that book many more times. You can't always take everything in the very first time you read it. Also, it was helpful for me to have the frequent reminders within the book to take on board the ideas and techniques within it. It encouraged me anew, each time I read it, to stop feeling down and negative and to push out any worries or concerns in my mind.

I truly believed that the contents of the book were highly valuable and relevant to me, to such an extent that if there was anyone else whom I felt could benefit from the book and seemed interested in the ideas, I would share my copy of the book with them. I started looking for more books filled with similar strategies.

Since reading that, I have read over 200 other books and have listened to thousands of hours of audio books on a wide variety of topics, including self-help, human development, sociology and psychology. I prefer the term 'self-discovery' to self-help.

It isn't my intention to boast about how well read I am in this topic, but instead to profess upon you how beneficial it can be to constantly learn and develop on a journey to self-discovery through books, videos, podcasts, audio-books, seminars and so on, so that you're constantly keeping your mind open to new techniques. It empowers you to transform your life.

When you read a book or hear an audio-book, it is as if an idea has been planted within your brain. When you act upon any of the suggestions within the book, this allows growth and development. You do need to act, though. Actions are like food and water to the seeds, and they won't grow and develop without action. When you harvest your crop, it feels incredible. You'll be so proud of yourself and your achievements.

I do hope that this book has been useful to you, so

that you will re-read it and share the ideas within it (or the book itself) with friends and family so that they can benefit, too. I also want you to discover lots of other authors and speakers who discuss similar topics, so that you're constantly expanding your knowledge and skills, and gaining technical abilities to deal with any issue life throws at you.

You need to keep on learning to stay alive.

I was never a great reader when I was at school. I always used to opt for the easier route of summary books that told you the gist of what was happening.

I now have confidence and contentment; and II feel good about myself. I discovered that learning doesn't have to be just academic and rote memorization; learning can be learning more about who we are, daring to be who we are, and feeling stronger to be able to be less shy and express ourselves. In the first half of this book, you've learned a lot about yourself, and it can be tough to be totally honest. But, it's necessary so that you can move beyond this, to change and make great improvements to your life.

What Now?

I would like you to be committed to lifelong learning and development, so that you can constantly strive to develop and grow as a person - and be who you truly are.

Think about how exactly your life will be when

you're no longer shy. Who are you? What will you do? Where will you go? Is there a difference that you will make to the world?

We don't 'just' want to focus solely on becoming less shy, because there's more to life than that.

Life is short; there are no reruns or second chances with it. You don't want to live just a middling, average, run-of-the-mill life. You want your life to be extraordinary! I know that you have things that are very special about you that set you apart from other people. You are talented, you are able, and you have a gift that you could share with the world. Dare to be yourself. Dare to live life as you want to. You will constantly throughout life have people telling you how you 'should' be and you need to be who YOU want to be.

Be you - exactly as you are. You are you; you are special; you are perfect exactly as you are. Live a life that you're proud of. I believe you're capable of anything that you put your mind to.

Bonus

You have everything you need within this book to become less shy and express yourself fluently and with ease. If there are moments when you need to push yourself into action, you now know the countdown from 3 technique, which will force you into action.

Before this book ends, I wanted to share a final story with you. This transformed how I live my life, and I feel certain your life could be changed too.

When I was younger, my dad would drive me to school. This became a bit of a tradition. The journey was only approximately 12 minutes, and during that time, I felt I could talk to my dad about anything. This could be school, relationships, sport, politics, or life in general. It was a very open space, where I could say anything. My father was definitely an adult. He wasn't like one of my friends my age; but he was also my confidant.

When we reached the school gates, he would hand me some money to go towards lunch, give me a hug, and then say, "Be the best person you can be today!"

As I was growing up throughout my teenage years, this seemed like a warm and fond saying from my dad, but I hadn't fully realised the significance of the words.

A lot of time has passed since my school days. Life is challenging at times, with various hurdles in the way. I look back very fondly on that time spent with my Dad, and I have frequently thought of those words.

If we constantly strive each day to 'Be the best person we can be,' we need to be fully aware of who we truly are as people. We need to be thankful and appreciative for the good things in life that we have. We need to be calm and content. We need to be totally truthful to ourselves and others. If we make an error, we need to own up to it and try to resolve it. We need to keep humility, be as loving as possible, find new adventures to keep us challenged and intrigued, push ourselves beyond our comfort zones to stretch and grow, and we need to try to make a difference to other people's lives, too.

Thank you for reading this book and letting me try to help you on your journey to becoming less shy and having the ability to express yourself. I hope that there's at least one thing you can take away from this book that has made a difference to you. Please feel free to share the book with your friends and family so that it can help them to understand you better, and perhaps pass on some hints and tips to them, too.

Be the best YOU that you're able to, today and ever after.

Good luck and best wishes!

***